THE KETO OMAD DIET

How to combine the Ketogenic Diet with the One Meal A Day Intermittent Fasting Diet to Maximize Your Weight Loss

by

MARKUS WILKINSEN

Legal Notes

This document contains opinions and ideas of the author. It is sold for the purpose of providing helpful and reliable information; the publisher, author, and all other parties involved in the making of this document are not required to render any qualified services or advice.

The information provided herein is strictly for educational and entertainment purposes; any liability, in terms of inattention or otherwise, by any usage or abuse of any policies, processes, or directions contained within, is the solitary and utter responsibility of the reader.

The content and information contained in this book have been compiled from sources deemed reliable, and it is accurate to the best of the Author's knowledge, information, and belief. However, the Author cannot guarantee its accuracy and validity and cannot be held liable for any errors and/or omissions. Further, changes are periodically made to this book as and when needed. Where appropriate and/or necessary, you must consult a professional (including but not limited to your doctor, attorney, financial advisor or such other professional advisor) before using any of the suggested remedies, techniques, or information in this book.

Under no circumstances will any legal responsibility or blame be held against the publisher, author, or any other parties involved in the making of this document for any reparation, damages, or monetary loss due to the information herein, either directly or indirectly. This disclaimer applies to any loss, damages or injury caused by the use and application, whether directly or indirectly, of any advice or information presented, whether for breach of contract, tort, negligence, personal injury, criminal intent, or under any other cause of action.

You agree to accept all risks of using the information presented inside this book.

Permission is not granted to reproduce, duplicate, or transmit any part of this document in electronic or

Table of Contents

INTRODUCTION

The Ketogenic diet is currently one of the most popular weight loss diets today. Do a search on the internet and it is almost a certainty that you will see articles, blogs, books, and even videos on the keto diet.

The OMAD diet however, is not as well spread but just as effective. OMAD stands for "One Meal A Day" and it is a type of Intermittent Fasting diet that is just as effective as the keto diet. However, it is not about starving yourself thin.

The keto diet promotes low carb, high fat, high protein meals, while OMAD doesn't restrict what you eat but restricts you to one meal only, and within a certain timeframe each day.

When you consider these two diets, both the keto diet and the OMAD diet are individually demanding of your willpower and they also individually force your body to undergo a series of changes. Putting both of them together might seem even more taxing on your body. However, this is not the case.

With the right approach and understanding the ketogenic diet and the OMAD diet can not only be incorporated to work together but they actually make it easier for you to lose weight.

Eating one meal a day combined with the keto diet is possible and in fact many people do it with success; the keto diet and OMAD diet have a lot in common which encourages people to use the two diets together as you will learn in this book.

This is a major dietary change and your body will need to be able to adapt to it. Paired with the OMAD diet which has its own adaptations needed, you might want to consider introducing these changes one at a time especially because of the dietary restrictions of the keto diet.

This restricted diet alone is a challenge for many people to manage, as the adjustment period is complicated by the cravings you will experience for carbohydrates when starting out. While these will go away after a few days, your body will crave sugary carbohydrates because it is so used to using them to fuel your body with energy from sugar.

Keto and OMAD have a unique series of benefits worth exploring. If you are interested in trying either of these diet styles out, it is worth knowing why they work so well together and how keto can help with the OMAD diet.

So exactly what is the Ketogenic OMAD Diet? This book will teach you everything you need to know.

You will learn all you need to know about both these diets, how more powerful they become if you combine them, and how you can combine both of them to work to accelerate your weight loss.

The Keto OMAD Diet Is Not For You If...

If any of the above apply to you, then please put down this book. Your long term health and well-being is at risk.

You should not do Keto OMAD if:

- You are pregnant or breastfeeding
- You have a history of an eating disorder
- You have a history of a sleeping disorder
- You are underweight

Also you must consult a doctor first if:

- You have a long-term medical condition (e.g. cancer, diabetes, ulcerative colitis, epilepsy, anemia, liver, kidney or lung disease).
- You have a condition that affects your immune system.
- You are on medication.

Note that this book is not intended to replace the advice of a trained medical professional.

If you're still with me let's learn more about how the ketogenic diet and intermittent fasting with One Meal A Day can change the way you approach weight loss forever.

CHAPTER 1

The Ketogenic Diet

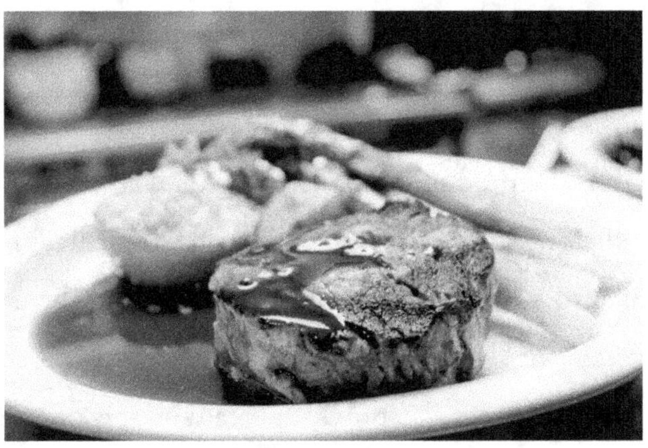

Ketogenic diet is a low carb, high protein, high fat diet. It is basically a diet designed to put the body in ketosis, a state in which the body burns fats to create ketones. These ketones are then used by the cells as energy for various cellular processes in place of glucose which is derived from carbohydrates.

Basics of the Ketogenic Diet

The diet is essentially promoting ketosis by limiting carbohydrate intake. This will drastically reduce the glucose absorbed from what you eat. This will cause the body to look for other energy sources, namely, the muscles and the stored body fats.

Ketosis encourages the body to burn its fat stores. The result is the production of ketone bodies which are by-products of fat breakdown. It is used by the cells as fuel, similar to how the cells use glucose. However, the main difference is that ketones do not need insulin to enter the cells. Ketones also provide a steady supply of energy over a longer period than glucose.

Generally, you should avoid all carb rich foods like bread, pasta, rice, legumes (peas, beans and lentils), corn, milk and refined sugar. The diet, however, does allow small amounts of carbs through starchy vegetables and fruits.

Your main goal is to change your macronutrient allowances. Your maximum carbohydrate intake should be limited to 30 grams a day. Some diet plans may allow 25 to 50 grams, depending on individual health conditions and health goals.

Fats should replace the carbs and make up the majority of your caloric intake, while proteins which are mainly from meat and dairy make up the rest of your diet.

On the ketogenic diet, you should aim for:

- 70 to 80% of daily calorie requirement from fats
- 20 to 25% of daily calorie requirement from proteins
- 5 to 10% of daily calorie requirement from carbohydrates.

If you need 2,000 calories per day, your meals should have:

- 1,400 to 1,600 calories from fats (155.6 grams to 177.8 grams)
- 400 to 500 calories from proteins (100 to 125 grams)

- 100 to 200 calories from carbohydrates (25 to 50 grams)

Carbs and Keto

While ketosis is the goal of the keto diet, restricting carbs is the safest way to achieve this. The question that most people have is "how many carbs can I take on the keto diet?"

For most people that is around 30 grams of carbs per day for 3 days. Commonly most guidelines for the keto diet recommend up to 60 grams a day. Generally carb intake on the keto diet has to be low in order to get our bodies into ketosis.

If you work out with high intensity training, or do a lot of physical activity then you could eat more carbs and not stop ketosis. This is due to your muscles using up the glycogen more quickly and in higher amounts. This is known as "carb cycling".

If you are like most of us who live sedentary lifestyles, then sticking to the 30 gram limit will help.

Additionally, you can follow these 3 guidelines to help you to reach ketosis:

1. Eat low-carb, low glycemic index foods

2. Avoid high-carb, high glycemic index foods

3. Choose low-carb alternatives

What is Ketosis?

Ketosis is a state in which the body runs on ketones instead of glucose which is derived from carbs. This state is induced if the body has very little intake of carbohydrates which means that there is less carbs for the body to convert into glucose.

The body will adapt to lack of carbohydrates and look for alternative fuel sources which will be the proteins stored in the muscles and the fats. Ketosis happens when the body breaks down fats and the products are converted into ketones.

The ketones are a steadier supply of energy unlike glucose. They enter the cells more easily and do not need insulin like glucose does. They're good brain fuel.

Some even argue that ketones are better energy sources for brain cells than glucose.

Reaching Ketosis

Restricting carbs to below 50 grams per day, boosting fat intake to 80% of your daily calories, and being moderate with protein is a sure way to reach ketosis. Once you are in ketosis, your body has made the switch from sugar burning to fat burning. There are three phases to how ketosis takes place in your body on a low-carb diet:

Phase I – Glycogen Depletion

In the first 1-3 days on a low-carb diet, your body turns to your liver and muscle glycogen to increase blood sugar levels. Glycogen is the stored form of glucose and that your body uses up within just a few days of low-carb eating.

Phase II – Fat Oxidation

When glycogen stores are used up, your body is forced to turn to its fat stores for energy production. Some of these fats are used for energy while others are converted into ketones. The reason your body makes ketones is that some cells (e.g. brain cells) cannot run on fatty acids and need alternative sources of energy. However, if your fat intake is high enough, your body will be using dietary fat for ketone production instead of using its fat stores.

Phase III – Ketone Utilization

It takes time for your body to adjust to the changes in fuel availability. Some people take longer to adapt to the ketogenic diet, while others seem to make the switch effortlessly. But around 2-4 weeks is an average for most. When your body starts utilizing ketones and oxidizing fat for energy, you have officially become keto adapted.

The 3 Types of Ketones

There are three main types of ketones found in our bodies.

Acetoacetate: This is the ketone that is first created. It has a role as a human metabolite, meaning that it is the product of metabolism. It can then be converted into either beta-hydroxybutyrate or acetone.

Acetone: Created spontaneously from the breakdown of acetoacetate. The production of acetone will increase as our bodies produce more ketones, and can be easily detectable on our breath when we are in ketosis.

Beta-hydroxybutyrate (BHB): This is the ketone that is used by our bodies for energy and it is the most abundant ketone found in our blood once we are in a state of ketosis. Exogenous ketone supplements are commonly based on beta-hydroxybutyrate and help you get back into ketosis when you eat too much carbs.

Keto Flu

In the process of reaching ketosis, you might experience some side effects. These are generally referred to as "keto flu." The symptoms are similar to a flu, and most people would experience fatigue, headaches, nausea, and cramps. Don't worry though, it's not a real flu and neither is it contagious. This is simply a result of fluid and electrolyte loss from glycogen depletion. These should last no more than a week, although most people report that from their experience it would last 3 to 5 days. Others may not even feel any of these side effects. Remember that our bodies are all different and we may experience this differently.

So what causes keto flu?

This is simply our bodies adapting to a major change in our diet. This change in diet causes a huge shock to the body. And because glycogen is stored with a large amount of water, when your body uses up glycogen it also uses up the water and electrolytes with it.

The solution to the keto flu is easy to treat. We just need to increase our fluid intake, especially with electrolyte drinks (such as sports drinks), and not over exert ourselves.

The Variations of the Keto Diet

Due to the different reasons that people go on the keto diet as well as their lifestyle and their goals, there are a few variations to the keto diet. Note that most of these variations have not been tested under laboratory conditions or studied by medical researchers.

Remember to consult with your doctor or nutritionist before adopting any of these diets.

Strict Keto Diet

This is also commonly referred to as the "keto therapy diet", or "therapeutic keto diet". This diet was created to help treat epileptic seizures and was published in Current Treatment Options in Neurology in 2008.

This version of the keto diet limits carbs very strictly. Your macros on the strict keto diet is:

- 90% of daily calorie requirement from fats

- 6% of daily calorie requirement from proteins

- 4% of daily calorie requirement from carbohydrates

Standard Keto Diet

This is the most common variation of keto used mainly for weight loss.

- 75% of daily calorie requirement from fats

- 20% of daily calorie requirement from proteins

- 5% of daily calorie requirement from carbohydrates

Cyclical Keto

Cyclical Keto follows the standard keto diet (above) but only for 5 or 6 days in a given week. Then for the other 1 or 2 days they eat normal amount of carbs in their meals.

This makes the diet a lot easier as it allows "cheat days" each week, allowing people to eat the foods that they have been missing. A caution however, is that the "cycling" part of cyclical keto should only be adopted once you have been on keto for a while and your body has adapted.

Lazy Keto

Lazy Keto, similar to cyclical keto, is designed to make keto more accessible to more people. The guidelines here are simple: Just count carbs. That's it.

Following the fat and protein requirements are complicated and most people would wrack their brains trying to figure out how much protein and fat a plate of food contains. The lazy keto solution then, is just to track your carbs and let the rest take care of itself.

It's hardly scientific but the results should be similar to regular keto. After all, controlling carbs is the biggest part of getting your body into ketosis.

How Long to Stay on Keto

It is generally accepted that the ketogenic diet works in the short term. There is enough evidence and medical research on this as an effective way to lose weight.

However, the expert opinion in the long term is uncertain. While there are critics who believe that there are long term effects that can be unhealthy, there are also others who believe that it can work in the long term.

Most nutritionists suggest that the maximum length of a keto diet should be 6 months, but most would suggest being on keto for 3 months at most. This is because removing carbohydrates as well as certain major food groups from your diet may lead to nutrient deficiencies.

However, the research on the long term effects of the keto diet is lacking. Most of the advice given by professionals regarding this is a very well educated guess, but it should not be ignored. After all it is better to be safe than sorry.

CHAPTER 2

The OMAD Diet

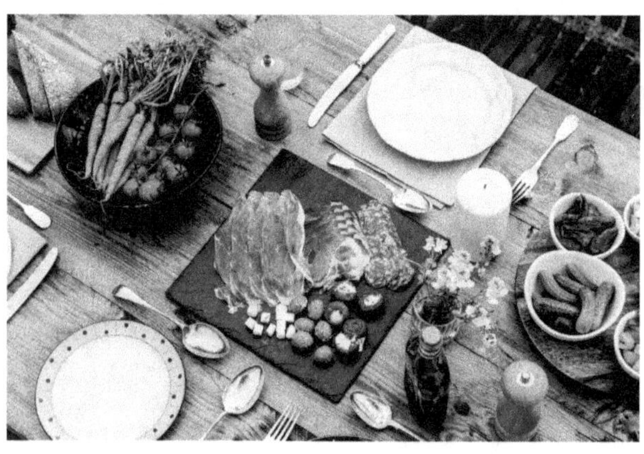

The One Meal a Day (OMAD) Diet is a weight loss method based on Intermittent Fasting. The main principles of this are regulating your meal frequency, and meal timing. This is a proven way that many people have used to lose body fat and keep it off. OMAD is also known as the 23:1 plan as people on this diet would fast for 23 hours and have an hour to eat their one meal.

Note that this is not a fad diet, nor is it a temporary weight loss solution.

Most diets are short term and result in a yo-yo effect where people actually lose weight but then they are unable to keep themselves off a pizza or chocolate bar. They end up caving in to their cravings, or they are unsatisfied with the weight loss that they have achieved. Either way, they end up giving up on their diet and some even gain more weight than they have lost while on a diet.

The issue is that these diets do not address the root cause of weight loss, which is to manage the circadian rhythm. This is done by timing exercise, meals and sleep which is managed when we stick to the rule of 4 "Ones" of the OMAD diet which will be covered in this chapter.

The reason the OMAD diet works is because it is a lifestyle and one that works for the long term because it is based in science.

Fasting strategies such as OMAD can be used as a tool to improve our lives. They are simple, yet effective. If you can follow the plan you will improve your health, energy, and well being. You do not have to count calories, worry about what you can or cannot eat, and mostly you do not have to feel guilty for cheat days.

Starting the OMAD Diet

While eating one meal a day may sound simple at first, there is a recommended approach to this diet. Like any other diet, the beginning of the switch in eating habits will require conscious effort to maintain, and you will need to build on this consistently in order to achieve long term success. When you are consistent in your daily eating habits, the diet starts to take effect and help you achieve the weight loss that you have set out for yourself.

The basis of the OMAD diet is the rule of 4 "Ones".

In essence, this means you should have:

1. One Hour

2. One Meal

3. One Plate

4. One Beverage

This rule helps you to maintain the discipline and have a structure to your diet. Many people have found this method to work best for weight loss, as well as maintaining a long term healthy lifestyle. So how do you follow the Rule of 4 Ones?

One Hour

When starting the one meal a day diet, you need to choose a four hour window to eat. This can be any four hours you want, but make sure it will best fit into your schedule as it would be best to stay consistent with the eating window.

Once you have chosen your four hour window, you should allow yourself one hour for your meal so you have sufficient time to enjoy your food which can include a beverage of your choice. When the hour is up, there should be no more calorie intake until the next eating window.

When choosing your eating window, it might take some time to figure out how to choose the best one to fit your situation, but maintaining a structure will make all the difference in your weight loss journey.

One Meal

Each day, you will have a 4 hour eating window but you should only give yourself 1 hour in those 4 hours to eat. In that one hour, you will have only one meal.

In the OMAD diet, there should be no small meals or cheat hours where you can eat snacks or junk food.

The only exception to this is for protein shakes taken post workout. If you do workout, these protein shakes are necessary to fuel your body with protein.

One Plate

Since you are restricted to one meal, it may be tempting to pile on whatever you want in your one hour window. When you are eating your one meal, it's important to understand what is going on your plate and ensure that there is a balance of nutrients, proteins, and carbohydrates.

It is recommended to incorporate a serving of vegetables, carbohydrates (potatoes, rice, or bread), protein and fats (from meats), and a serving of fruits. The caloric intake for most people during OMAD is around 1,500 Kcal.

An average sized plate could actually hold two servings of meals so it is important that you make an informed choice of what goes onto your plate and not overeat during your one meal.

<u>One Beverage</u>

During your meal, you should allow yourself to have one beverage of your choice. This can be anything you crave, from beer to a soda, or anything else you want. This serves as a perk me up to boost your mood. The OMAD diet is not about depriving yourself, it is just a structured way to approach your food and drink intake.

Taking a drink with a caloric count can also help you to get your calories required for the day, but you should keep yourself to one serving.

Apart from this, you should continue to hydrate yourself by drinking water throughout the day. You do not have to limit your intake of water. Tea and coffee can also be drunk at any time, as it may help to suppress your hunger.

What to Expect When Starting OMAD

When starting out on OMAD diets, the most common thing that people experience is hunger, as one would expect, so know that you are not alone. This is most likely an issue of body conditioning that you will have to battle the first few weeks. You may not actually be hungry, but because you have been eating several times a day, your body has been conditioned to expect food every few hours. This is something that everyone on the OMAD diet would have to push through.

While this will vary from person to person, a "fasting headache" is common for the first few weeks at least.

This is triggered by a combination of low blood sugar, dehydration, and possibly lack of sleep. The trick is to stay hydrated throughout your fast as it will help to ease the headaches and hunger pangs.

The brain is 75% water and is very sensitive to dehydration, and produced histamines to ration and conserve water when faced with a shortage. It is these histamines that cause headaches as well as fatigues; they are a signal that we need to drink more water. Keep in mind that this discomfort will end once your body gets used to your new eating schedule and the lack of intermittent snacks throughout the day.

Another good way of keeping hunger at bay is to keep yourself busy with work or distracting yourself with other activities. This will help you keep your mind off food. Consciously staying away from the kitchen or the pantry will also help as you will not be constantly seeing and smelling food to whet your appetite when it is not your meal time. Out of sight, out of mind.

Once your mind has been disciplined to eat only meal a day, your body will adjust eventually.

Three types of OMAD

While the OMAD diet may be simple and uncomplicated, there are three main ways in which it is practiced.

OMAD with Caloric Restriction

This form of OMAD is usually used by people looking to lose weight fast. This variation puts a limit on the total amount of calories, and then have you consume it all in one meal. To figure out how many calories to set for yourself, you should check your Total Daily Energy Expenditure (TDEE).

Be careful when restricting your calories on a strict fasting diet, especially if you are also implementing keto.

Going too low may cause dizziness, fatigue, and lethargy in the short run. If this happens, you should consider breaking your fast to eat something rather than suffer through it.

In the long term, constant caloric restriction may cause damage to your body.

OMAD without Caloric Restriction

This form of OMAD does not restrict calories. You can have as much food as you want in one sitting.

A study published in The American Journal of Clinical Nutrition in 2009 found that reduced meal frequencies without caloric restriction was effective in weight loss. Most middle aged adults in the study experienced fat loss and weight loss

Usually the restriction here is on the one plate, and one hour. Healthy food choices and a balanced meal are also highly recommended. This is much less complicated than restricting your calories.

If you are implementing keto as well, it is common for dieters to use this form of OMAD with the "lazy keto" strategy to get the benefits of both with the least amount of fuss.

OMAD without Restriction

This form of OMAD has restrictions only on your eating window. You have one hour to consume whatever you want. That includes fried chicken, burgers, pizza etc. If you are on keto as well, remember that your food choices still have to limit carbs and favor fats.

You should still make healthy food choices, but with this variation it is not something that is monitored.

How OMAD is Practiced

While OMAD is "One Meal A Day" and it is supposed to be a lifestyle change, there are also variations to how often people go OMAD. Sure, there are people that practice this every day and make it work.

Practically though, there are people who only go OMAD occasionally while they practice other methods of Intermittent Fasting. There are also people who only practice OMAD every alternate day, or only on weekends.

The key here is to make your diet and fasts work with your schedule. To make any diet work in the long term, it should not be stressful and it should not make you miserable. If you have to cancel nights out with friends, stop working out, or if fasting and meal timings affect your job then you're doing it wrong. You shouldn't need to force a diet.

To make OMAD work in the long run you need to:

Get Sufficient Nutrients

Because you only have one meal a day, you need to get your nutrients, vitamins, and calories in one sitting. This becomes more important if you are maintaining OMAD over a long period of time.

Having a healthy diet with the right nutrients and calories will help you feel better about your diet and help you maintain your daily activity levels. Choosing "real" , a.k.a. unprocessed foods, will help reduce the preservatives and chemicals you consume and increase your nutrient intake.

Have a Positive Relationship with Food

A common problem with people who practice any fasting diet is that it can easily promote an unhealthy relationship with food. Since they have to stay fasted, it is easy to start perceiving food as bad. If you have struggled with eating disorders in the past this can exacerbate any food habits that are harmful.

OMAD should be used to build a healthy relationship with food by making informed choices and enjoying your meals. Fasting should not be punishment for something that you ate.

Be Kind to Yourself

Remember that our bodies are all unique. You have your own considerations, circadian rhythms, dietary restrictions, and medical issues (if any). Any diet that you undertake will have to take all that into consideration. Choose a diet that fit your lifestyle, and works for your body.

There might be days when you need more calories. You could be planning a lot of physical activity, have a more stressful day at work, a bad night's sleep, or just under the weather. In these situations it may not be a good idea to fast. It would do your overall health and wellbeing a lot of good if you were to plan around that. When you have adapted to your diet, remember to listen to your body.

The purpose of any diet is to make you healthier, make you feel better, and allow you a better quality of life. If you ever feel unwell, you should stop your diet and consult with a doctor or medical professional.

CHAPTER 3

How the Keto OMAD Diet Speeds Up Weight Loss

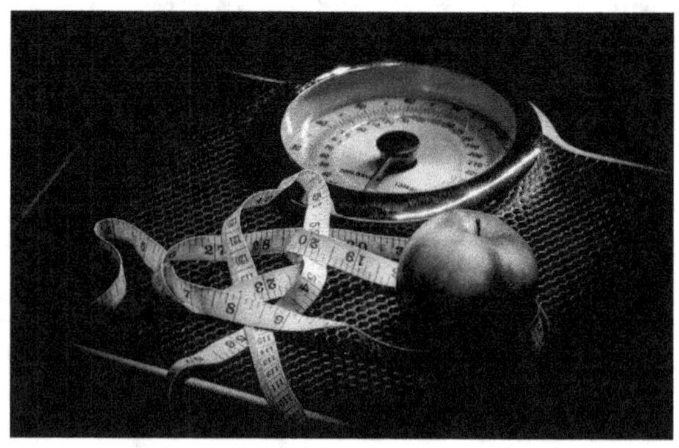

OMAD brings the body into a fat-burning state. The keto diet enhances that process and drives the body to use ketones instead being of glucose-dependent.

OAMD, generally speaking, is just fasting and does not necessarily restrict the kind of food you can eat, even sugar-rich foods and junk foods can lead to weight loss if you eat once a day (although it might not be the best choice). It works just as it is. But by adding the keto diet to the OMAD diet, high carb foods are removed to further support the fat-burning process initiated by the fasting period.

In fact, fasting is commonly used by people who follow the ketogenic diet in order to speed up ketosis although it is not necessary. A study published in the Journal of Child Neurology in 2002 found that both fasting and the ketogenic diet led to ketosis in the same timeframe. However, putting the two together hastens the process and additionally it reduces the risk of hypoglycemia and electrolyte imbalances that are the risks of fasting and keto respectively.

That's right, the Keto OMAD diet is scientifically proven to be more effective than keto or OMAD alone.

An Alternative to Calorie Restriction

While some versions of OMAD does have a calorie restriction, in general the rule of 4 "ones" does not limit your calories directly. Similarly, the keto diet only limits your carb intake to not more than 50 grams a day but does not limit your calories. It just promotes low carb and replacing carbs with more fats and moderate amounts of proteins.

While you can also restrict calories to improve the effects of both these diets, the real benefit is in making healthy choices using both the guidelines of the OMAD and keto diets together.

Combining the two, you eat one keto meal that is high in fat and low in carb, then fast. Why is this much better, healthier way to manage weight and body fat?

Most other weight loss programs restrict calories, some to the extreme. This is actually counterproductive. Weight loss may be rapid but it's much more difficult to stay in this type of diet. Results are also short-lived. Worse, all the weight lost returns and much more.

Too much calorie restriction is actually riskier on your health, too. Here's why:

1. Slows down metabolism

If you feed the body with too little calories, it will compensate by slowing down metabolism. Calorie restriction can slows down calorie burning by up to

23%. This slowed metabolism can continue even after the low-calorie diet is discontinued.

Many researchers believe that this continued slowdown of metabolism is the main reason why people regain the weight they lost early in the low-calorie diet. This is also a main factor why people gain more weight when they stop their low-calorie diet.

The body reduces its energy consumption to conserve its energy stores aka fat. That also leads to slower fat burning.

2. Muscle loss

This is a result of slowed metabolism. Muscle loss more likely occurs if the low-calorie diet is also low in proteins. This is common as people on low-calorie diets tend to stay off meats thinking that the fats in them are bad. Not having enough exercise while on low-calorie diets also promote muscle loss.

3. Fatigue

Of course, if you are not eating enough, you have little energy. You easily become fatigued. Add the slowed metabolism and it will be difficult to perform daily tasks, much less get some exercise.

This becomes worse if the calorie-restricted diet has very low carbohydrate contents.

4. Nutrient deficiencies

Eating very little also runs the risk of having nutrient deficiencies. Calorie restrictions result in inadequate intake of vitamin B12, iron and folate. If the deficiencies are not addressed soon, it can lead to extreme fatigue and anemia.

Limiting calories also often means limiting eating foods rich in these nutrients:

- Proteins- usually from omitting foods like meats, dairy, fish, nuts and seeds

- Calcium- usually from omitting foods like dairy, milk and leafy greens

- Thiamine and biotin- usually from omitting foods like eggs, legumes, dairy, whole grains, seeds and nuts

- Magnesium- usually from omitting foods like leafy greens, nuts and whole grains

Why OMAD with the Keto Diet Makes Sense

The extreme fasting window of at least 20 hours when on the OMAD diet will often trigger ketosis. This is true even if you have eaten carbohydrates since they will be used up as energy in a few hours. After that, your body will begin to go into ketosis and burn fatty acids.

So fasting can promote ketosis but it will usually take 18 to 24 hours for this to happen. This is why more people prefer going on long fasts 1-2 times a week to keep their bodies in ketosis. However, long fasts are challenging for many people.

Short fasts do not produce enough ketosis. Moreover, weight lost during these short fasts is generally from depletion of glycogen stores in the liver. When the body metabolizes glycogen, it also losses 3-4 grams of water per gram of glycogen used. Hence, the criticism is that most of the weight lost during short fasts is from water loss, not fat loss.

When glycogen stores fall and very little glucose enters the body, the body starts to turn to its other energy stores- fats and proteins. The proteins are stored in the muscles and the fats are stored in many places in the body such as the thighs and belly area.

The body metabolizes its proteins in the muscles first. Proteins are broken down into amino acids. These amino acids are then converted into glucose through a process known as gluconeogenesis.

However, losing proteins is dangerous for the body. Losing even a third of the body's protein stores result in a number of health and medical issues. Hence, it will turn to the fat stores for energy.

At some point in your fast, usually 2-3 days of not eating, fats are broken down into glycerol and fatty acids. These are converted in the liver into ketone bodies. These ketones bodies are used by the brain and the muscles, including the visceral muscles of all our organs.

However, the brain cannot function on ketones alone. It still needs a small amount of glucose, about 30 g a day to function normally. If you are not eating, glucose will have to come from protein breakdown in the muscles.

Since losing too many proteins can be dangerous, this is where ketogenic diet becomes very helpful in combination with OMAD fasting.

Here are some things you need to keep in mind while on Keto OMAD:

1. We cannot fast safely and healthily for more than 24 hours, more than 1-2 times a week. Otherwise, we risk experiencing the abovementioned conditions.

2. In order to get the body to burn fats, we need it to deplete its glycogen stores so it will turn to other energy stores- muscles and fats.

3. Losing muscles is not a good thing.

4. The brain needs small amounts of glucose a day, even if it can function quite well on ketones.

The Ketogenic OMAD diet has an answer for these:

Eating one meal a day helps to kick start our liver into using our glycogen stores first. This would put our bodies into ketosis the first time we go on the fast.

This process is then extended by eating ketgenic meals that are low-carb, and high protein, high fat. When we reduce our carbohydrate intake to 50 grams or less our bodies continue to deplete its glycogen stores. Once depleted, the body turns to muscles and fats for fuel.

Since muscle loss is something we want to avoid, we prevent it with meals that include proteins. Hence, the body digests these proteins and turns them into fuel instead of the proteins in the muscles. If any proteins in the muscles were metabolized, proteins in the diet can be used to replace them.

Ketogenic meals also contain small amounts of glucose. This helps the brain get its daily dose of glucose for optimum functioning.

All the while, you get to lose a lot of weight rapidly. As you use glycogen stores, you lose excess water. As the body continues to function with little glucose from meals and from glycogen metabolism, it will turn to its fat stores.

You burn fats, you don't starve yourself and most importantly, your body gets the macronutrients it needs. Moreover, since you are not removing any food groups in your meals while on the keto diet you still provide the body with the micronutrients such as vitamins and minerals it needs for its metabolic and cellular processes.

Keto and the Side Effects of OMAD

Like any diet, OMAD has its side effects. However, some of them can be mitigated by switching to the keto diet.

Keto OMAD Reduces Insulin Resistance

Insulin is an essential hormone in order to get glucose out of the blood and into the cells. If the glucose remains in the blood, this can accumulate and lead to potentially dangerous high blood sugar levels. The high levels persist and become a chronic condition. This can lead to problems such as diabetes, cardiovascular problems, high blood pressure and organ damage.

One condition that can lead to chronically high blood sugar levels is insulin resistance.

This is a condition wherein the cells are no longer responsive to the presence of insulin. This unresponsiveness results in glucose in the blood unable to enter the cells. It remains in the blood and create chronically high blood sugar levels.

A short-term response is an increase in insulin production and secretion by the pancreas. As the insulin resistance persists, the pancreas will not be able to hold out any longer. It will eventually give up with all the blood sugar it has to address.

The pancreas gets damaged and the problem gets worse. There is now high blood sugar with high insulin levels in the blood.

Diseases start to develop such as type 2 diabetes. It can also lead to serious chronic conditions such as:

- High cholesterol and elevated triglycerides

- Heart disease and high blood pressure

- Stroke

- Non-alcoholic fatty liver disease and colorectal cancer

- Cancer

- Gout

- Alzheimer's disease

- Polycystic ovary syndrome

Going on a ketogenic diet helps to prevent or reverse insulin resistance. One of the main ways is by reducing the amount of carbohydrates in the diet. This alone can improve several health markers:

- High blood pressure

- Elevated blood sugar

- Excess body fat around your waist

- Abnormal cholesterol levels

Keto OMAD Reduces Cravings & Hunger Pangs

Cravings and hunger are common issues during a fast. This happens when we get insufficient food, or we do not choose the right type of foods to eat. A bowl of ice cream might meet your fat and caloric needs, but it is also high in sugars and will cause a "crash" when the calories are burned. Eating a whole chicken however, will make you feel full. It is satiating.

A study published by the Texas Tech University compared the effect of high fat meals on the satiety hormone and found that different fats affected a subjective measure of fullness. When we eat fat, it helps to regulate appetite through the release of hormone and it also affects our gastric function.

What this means is that omeals that have a higher amount of saturated or polyunsaturated fat help you feel full for a longer amount of time compared to foods that contain monounsaturated fats or no fats whatsoever.

Cravings is different from hunger and it is the body's response to low blood sugar levels. This can intensify during fasts. By eating fats on a keto diet during the eating window, blood sugar levels are more constant. There is research that has shown that people on a keto diet experienced lower levels of cravings for carbs or sweets as compared to people on a low fat diet.

On the ketogenic diet, your cells are receiving a constant supply of energy through ketones which suppresses ghrelin, the hunger hormone. This helps you to get through your fasting period.

CHAPTER 4

Benefits of the Keto OMAD Diet

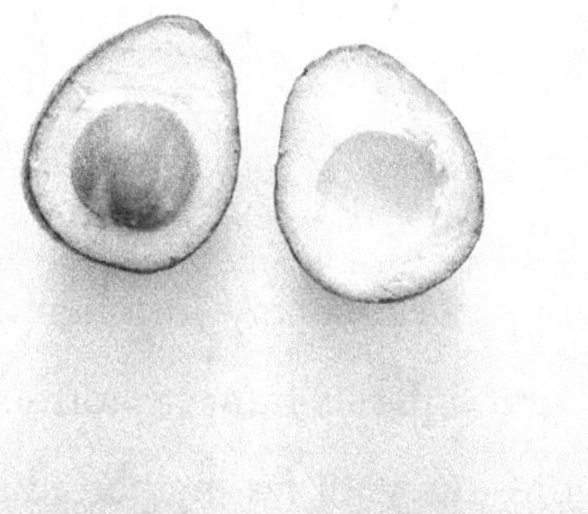

With the Keto OMAD diet, weight loss can seem counter intuitive. It prescribes eating one huge meal that is high fat, high protein, but low carb, all in one sitting. However, this diet does come with a whole lot of benefits beyond weight loss.

In this chapter, you will learn some of these benefits you will experience when you switch to a Keto OMAD diet.

There are a few studies that found that a ketogenic diet to be helpful in improving the health of your heart and the blood vessels by lowering the amount of cholesterol in the blood.

A study from Kuwait University found that the keto diet helped to increase the amount of the good type of cholesterol in the body called HDL or high density lipoprotein. As a result, levels of bad cholesterol called LDL (low density lipoprotein) went down significantly. They also found that ketogenic diet led to a significant reduction in both body mass index and body weight.

Fasting also has a positive impact on cholesterol. A 2012 study on cholesterol by AIM-HIGH Investigators showed that LDL (bad cholesterol) is reduced when fasting by up to 25%.

This is alongside other benefits such as reduced body weight and decreased waist size, as well as preserving HDL (good cholesterol) levels.

These effects can have a great impact towards protecting the heart and blood vessels against problems like atherosclerosis and heart attacks and this happens because the body switches from burning sugar, to burning our fat reserves when fasting and on keto.

Blood Pressure Control

A study published in Nutrition and Healthy Aging has found that fasting has reduced blood pressure by up to 7% in a number of individuals who participated in clinical studies. While the sample size is small, it does show promise.

Coupled with the weight loss benefits, and improved cholesterol, a reduction in blood pressure all contributes to a reduction in the risk of heart disease.

Reverse/Prevent Insulin Resistance

Insulin resistance is often linked to excessive intake of high carb meals. When we eat, insulin brings these sugars to our cells that are stored as fat.

Diabetes often results when the body has too much fat stores, the cells are insulin resistant and there is a continuous daily overload of glucose form food. This leads to overworking the liver, pancreas and cells in dealing with the massive influx of glucose at every meal or snack.

When we do not snack between meals insulin levels will drop and fat cells will start to release the sugar that they have stored. Therefore, by cutting down on our blood sugar, insulin levels are reduced and our bodies will start to burn fat.

When on the ketogenic diet, you significantly reduce your carb intake to a small 25 to 50 grams a day. Compared to an average of up to 100 grams when not on keto, this reduction gives the body a break from trying to catch up with glucose control.

Keto OMAD also burns fat which makes our cells less resistant to insulin. This prevents sugar spikes and the accompanying sugar crashes that come along with it.

Better Blood Glucose Control

Blood glucose levels is the main marker for diabetes. When it spikes it can lead to long term complications such as eye disease, kidney problems, stroke, and cardiovascular diseases.

When on the fasting, you eat less carbs, you cut back on sugar, and you stop snacking outside of your eating window. All this put together gives a much better blood glucose control as compared to when you are not fasting.

However, fasting alone may cause unstable blood sugar. It drops when we fast, and then spikes sharply when we have our meals. Especially so if we eat a high carb meal and it intensifies any cravings that we may have.

By switching the Keto OMAD, we eat more fats and stay in ketosis through fasting and a keto diet, our bodies get a break from the glucose-driven processes.

Our blood sugar levels are more constant. Spikes are not as frequent, leading to more consistent energy levels. Also, our livers and pancreas get a break from the years of processing carbs, giving them a chance to return to optimal levels.

The obvious benefit of Keto OMAD is the weight loss that comes from sticking to the diet. By limiting yourself to one meal, one plate, and one beverage in one hour (the 4 "Ones" Rule), you are limiting your caloric intake. Snacks and other junk food have a large amount of calories that we are not aware of, and cutting them out helps us to lose weight and keep it off.

Most people will cut back up to 1,000 calories a day by staying away from the vending machine, potato chips, and chocolate. This can quickly shed up to a pound a week if maintained. If you don't eat for longer periods, your body gets a chance to burn some of its fat stores leading to further weight loss.

While other diets result in losing water weight resulting in dehydration, the OMAD Diet encourages you to constantly hydrate to stave off hunger headaches and fatigue. This means that any weight loss is truly fat loss rather than just dehydration.

Weight loss also happens with the decrease in insulin. Fasting reduces the amount of glucose the body absorbs from food. In response, the pancreas reduces the amount of insulin it produces and releases.

If you manage to stick to the diet plan and consistently exercise discipline in what and when you eat, it becomes a lifestyle change that sticks with you for good.

Burn Fat

Both the OMAD and keto diet individually promote fat burning without intentionally cutting back on caloric intake. No calorie counting, no food weighing, no special meal preps.

You can enjoy eating your favorite foods that are keto approved while burning fats. Fat loss continues when you enter the fasting period. This same burning process continues even after you have broken the fast and entered your next eating period.

When on the Keto OMAD diet, you ideally want to be burning fat as an energy source and the fasting period of your diet is a great way for burning body fat. When you are sleeping the body naturally gets into a fasted state where it automatically switches to a fat burning mode, and fasting prolong this natural fasting state. When you wake up and begin eating, your body produces insulin and starts to use the carbohydrates you consume as energy instead of fat.

By adding keto meals during the eating window, the fat-burning process stimulated during the fasting period is maintained. Hence, more fat loss results.

People lose 7% of their body weight with this combination compared to people who eat unhealthy carb-laden foods (only 3% of their body weight).

More Muscle Gain

Fasting for 24 hours does not lead to muscle loss. On the contrary, it increases the amount of human growth hormone (HGH) by as much as 1,300% in women and 2,000% in men. This HGH plays a key role in the muscle building process.

Higher HGH levels can boost muscle gain and slow down muscle loss. Higher levels of HGH also results in lower body fat, better bone mass and increased lean body mass.

Faster Recovery

Aside from muscle mass and body fat, HGH also helps in muscle recovery. HGH supports protein synthesis in the muscles. This process speeds up the recovery by speeding up repair of damaged or inflamed muscle tissues. This is helpful as it promotes faster recovery from intense workouts or after an injury, thereby reducing downtime.

Drives Autophagy

Autophagy is a natural body process that makes sure tissues are well maintained. Autophagy means self-eating. Cells "eat" old or damaged cells to make room for new ones. This is like spring cleaning that helps tissues function at optimum levels.

This process helps to lower inflammation. It also contributes to longevity, as cells are continually renewed.

Researchers found that autophagy occurs most significantly in the brain. Dr Mark Mattson, a Neurology Professor at John Hopkins University has found that fasting increases the growth and development of brain cells and nerve tissues.

Additionally, fasting has also shown to reduce inflammation in the brain which can lead to Alzheimer's and other neurodegenerative disorders.

This is in line with what other people who fast have reported in terms of increased concentration, and better memory. This also results in being more mentally stable and alert during daily tasks.

Fasting periods promote increased amounts of a protein called BDNF. This protein is found in the brain. It improves memory and learning by promoting the formation of new neural pathways. This makes the brain work more efficiently.

Reduced Appetite

A keto meal provides a more steady supply of energy for the cells to use. If the cells have enough energy they need, you won't feel hungry.

Fats are more filling and take longer for our bodies to process compared to carbohydrates. Add a moderate protein intake and appetite can be suppressed for hours as our meals are slowly digested and absorbed.

Ketosis also promotes the suppression of ghrelin. This is an appetite regulating hormone. Low levels mean less hunger.

Improved Digestive System

Since you are eating only one meal a day, your digestive system isn't as overworked as before. If you reduce highly processed and fatty foods, digestive issues will be reduced even further.

If you have irritable bowels or other gastrointestinal issues, the Keto OMAD diet can help because you will not constantly be trying to process food in your gut. Gradually, you will feel better after meals.

But do remember to take high fiber vegetables to help with digestion.

Improved Immune System

There are many reports of people getting sick less often, and having more energy with Keto OMAD due to an improved diet. Many researchers have found that fasting may also reduce the risk of chronic diseases, including heart diseases.

When we stop eating and focus on resting, this reduces the stress on our internal systems. The energy we use to digest our food can instead be used for boosting our immune systems, our cognition, and other brain and body functions.

Drinking water while the body is fasting also allows our digestive system to flush out any micro organisms resulting in a better regulated immune system which means that we are healthier eating one meal a day.

Reduced Inflammation

Going on a fast daily helps in reducing oxidative stress on the cells. It also helps reduce the amounts of body-wide inflammatory markers.

Low inflammation helps the body perform better. It also contributes to longevity.

A More Positive Relationship With Food

The Keto OMAD diet when followed, can change a person's psychological approach to food.

People on the Keto OMAD diet have a healthier relationship with food, enjoying whatever they want instead of having secret "taboo" foods that they avoid only to binge on.

Counter intuitively, binge eating is also less likely to occur since the diet is about consistency. With the variety of food open to dieters, people are less likely to restrict themselves for long periods only to go wild on what they want to eat.

The Keto OMAD diet only restricts carbs, but otherwise promotes eating a regular amount at a regular time. People have reported that they are less likely to want to eat anything and everything, but have a better relationship with food through this diet.

Part of having a healthier approach to food is also enjoying food more. People on Keto OMAD have shared that they appreciate the taste of food more. They savor each bite that they take, and are able to enjoy exploring new spices and cooking styles in their diet.

Better Productivity

Usually, our bodies rely on the food we eat to give us energy by converting carbohydrates to sugar and then breaking it down. When we deprive ourselves of food for a long period like 23 hours, our blood sugar levels drop, and as a result insulin levels drop as well.

Our bodies then learn to look for an alternative source of energy, and turns to the fat we store.

Since we only eat once a day, our metabolism changes. When using fat instead of food as energy, fat needs to be slowly digested and sent to the liver for processing. This process happens steadily over time, and unlike eating does not have spikes in our blood sugar, or our metabolism.

With the use of coffee and tea, you can still use caffeine as a source of energy, as well as to trick your stomach into thinking you have eaten even though you have not.

A Lifestyle Change

Although it is called a "diet", Keto OMAD is actually a lifestyle change and brings with it many benefits.

Discipline is a huge factor in succeeding with the Keto OMAD diet, and it can be difficult at times to deal with the discomfort and the hunger, especially in the initial stages. This is a long term thing, to maintain the self discipline not just for a day, or a week, but for life.

CHAPTER 5

Side Effects of the Keto OMAD Diet

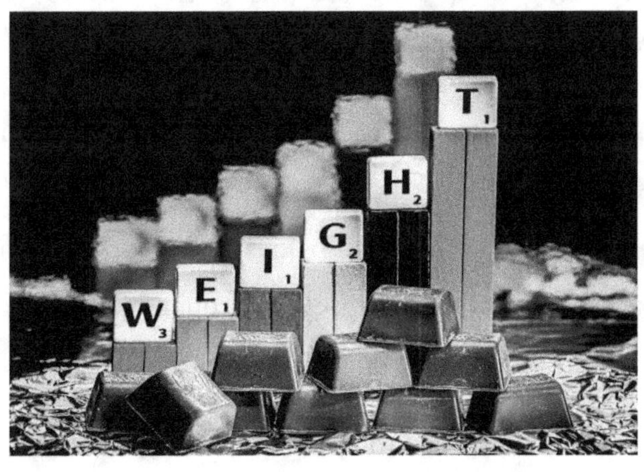

Every diet requires discipline, but OMAD more so than others. Deciding to embark on an OMAD Diet may also require you to decide in advance how much you are willing to commit to it. OMAD Diets are extremely effective, only if it is properly followed and maintained.

Only by following the 4 "Ones" Rule, and properly training your mind and body to overcome hunger pangs will you succeed. Going keto and eating more fats and protein helps with that somewhat. Remember that it is possible to achieve your weight loss goals that you set out for yourself, but it all depends on your dedication to the diet.

That being said, there are also some risks to Keto OMAD that you would have to be aware of.

There are serious risks for people with preexisting medical conditions such as diabetes. Diabetics suffer from low blood sugar, also known as hypoglycemia, and need to eat meals regularly throughout the day to avoid any serious side effects.

Pregnancy may also affect your decision to switch to a Keto OMAD diet. As pregnant women in their second and third trimesters (basically after 3 months of pregnancy) need to consume extra calories. While medical research in this area is still inconclusive, it is not recommended by most doctors to fast while pregnant as it can lead to complications like low birth weight of the child.

If you have suffered from eating disorders, it is also not recommended to try Keto OMAD. It is not worth sacrificing your mental health over your diet. Every time you fast, you are actively helping your eating disorder to take over your life.

In any case it is advisable to consult a doctor before beginning a Keto OMAD Diet.

Eating one meal a day can also have physical side effects such as weakness, exhaustion, and a lack of focus. Physical symptoms such as extreme hunger, weakness, fatigue, and being unable to concentrate may also appear in some people.

Hydration is important in dealing with most of these, but it is also important to consider your own personality. If you are unable to stick with the plan of the 4 "Ones" Rule and go full OMAD, you might want to consider other diets.

Here's what you can expect during the initial phases of the Keto OMAD diet.

When the body goes into the ketogenic state, side effects are usually felt. Some of these side effects are just part of the process of getting used to using ketones instead of glucose as fuel. Some go away after a few days. Some side effects may need a little management to reduce the severity.

The OMAD diet also comes with its own side effects. Oftentimes, these are just part of the body's transition from depending on glucose from meals to burning glycogen stores and fat stores for energy.

These side effects can be managed to make your diet more comfortable especially during the initial phase.

Frequent Urination

Hydrating is important but it will also make you urinate more often. You will have to make sure you have good access to the bathroom for this. You cannot reduce your water intake as it helps keep the side effects and risks for negative effects of fasting low.

Urinating is one of the main ways the body gets rid of waste and excess compounds. During the early stages of being in the ketogenic state, the body starts to burn the excess stored glycogen in the liver. This usually happens during the first 2 days of the ketogenic diet.

As a side effect, water retained in the tissues is also released. This excess water is brought to the kidneys for excretion.

This is the reason why most people on the ketogenic diet experience increased frequency of urination during the first few days. Some usually experience them for the first 2 days. Some might be longer, depending on how much excess water is retained and how much excess glycogen is being burned.

This side effect usually resolves in a few days as the body adjusts to the ketogenic state. Frequency of urination also returns to normal once the body does not burn through its extra glycogen stores.

Drowsiness and Dizziness

This often occurs as a side effect of increased urination. Urine is mostly water but also contains dissolved minerals. This includes sodium, magnesium and potassium.

These minerals play important roles in fluid balance as well as many other important processes. When the levels of these minerals drop because of frequent urination, it creates an imbalance.

As a result, fatigue, drowsiness and dizziness are felt.

Losing minerals is not a good thing. Low potassium levels, in particular, can lead to muscle weakness, fluid imbalances and, if severe, problems with cardiovascular functions.

Hence, it is important to replenish lost minerals, especially during the early days of the keto diet.

Add foods rich in minerals. Some of the best potassium sources are:

- Avocados
- Leafy greens
- Dairy
- Broccoli

- Fish, poultry and meats

Adding a little bit salt in meals replenishes lost sodium. Some people may have some reservations about adding more salt as it can be bad for the body. However, if on a keto diet with less than 60 grams of carbohydrate intake a day, lost salt must be replenished.

It is advisable to check with a doctor before increasing salt intake for those who are on high blood pressure medications. There might be a few necessary adjustments to how much salt can be added and the dosage of the medications to keep things in balance.

For magnesium, taking 400 mg magnesium citrate can help. Take the supplement before going to bed. There are also a few magnesium-rich foods that can be added into meals to keep magnesium levels normal. However, magnesium supplements not only add more of the minerals per tablet than per food serving, it can also help alleviate some of the other side effects of keto.

Hunger

This is expected as you will be changing your eating schedule. We have all grown up to eating 3 main meals-breakfast, lunch and dinner- with a snack in the morning and another in the afternoon.

Feelings of hunger are regulated by the hormone ghrelin. Higher levels of ghrelin make us feel hungry. Incidentally, ghrelin levels peak around breakfast, lunch and dinner, specifically during times you have been eating these meals on a regular basis.

Ghrelin levels are partially controlled by food intake.

For example, if you are used to eating breakfast at 6AM, your ghrelin levels adapts and peaks every day at 6AM. If you are used to eating breakfast at 10AM, that's also when your ghrelin levels peak.

During the first few fasts, ghrelin levels continue peaking at its regular times. Hence, you will feel hungry when peak times coincide with your fast. This will make it more challenging to go through the fast.

Days 3 to 5 will be the most challenging.

Once the body adjusts to the fasting schedules, there will be times when you have fasted long and come eating window, you still don't feel hungry.

Hunger during the first 1-2 weeks on OMAD can be managed by drinking a lot of water. This helps keep the belly full, mimicking the fullness when you eat. Hydrating also helps you be more alert and focused.

Drinking also address thirst. Often, thirst is felt as hunger.

Reduced Blood Sugar Levels

This is another common side effect during the early days of the keto diet. The body burns through its excess glycogen stores. This creates an artificial low blood sugar state.

The body is used to eating that brings in tons of glucose in the blood. The keto diet changes all that. In 1 to 2 days, all that changes. The body is thrown into a glucose-eating machine into a fat-burner. Glucose intake is drastically reduced from well over the average daily recommendation to ultra-low 60 grams.

Insulin levels will remain high, as if it is still dealing with loads of glucose from your meals. This results in low blood sugar levels.

It will take time for the body to adjust to being dependent on glucose for energy and rely on ketones from fat burning. The body will have to adjust to this and soon be able to regulate the amount of insulin it releases.

Low blood sugar is only temporary. Its symptoms include hunger, feeling tired all the time and feeling as if the body is shaky. These will go away so stay in keto.

Cravings

This is one of the most difficult challenges for many, whether on keto, OMAD, or any other weight loss diet. It's just too difficult to fight cravings

Cravings are a result of many factors. First, it's all in your mind. If you know you can't do something or eat something, all you can think of is that thing you are not supposed to do or eat.

Be prepared as the initial stage of ketogenesis will bring an intense craving for sugar. This transition period usually lasts for 1-2 days, or extended for about 3 weeks. On OMAD this would be amplified for some people.

When you are fasting, you know you won't eat for hours and yet your mind is filled with thoughts of food. Cravings start to be felt. These cravings are oftentimes for sugary, carbohydrate-rich foods. This is because the body is looking for a glucose hit for many reasons.

First, it feels threatened. The body thinks it is being starved. In response, it heightens its desire for food a.k.a. cravings in order to supply its energy needs. The body is not very keen on metabolizing its stores. It's quite a stingy hoarder when it comes to glucose. No wonder it's easy to pack in fats.

However, you are not starving your body. You are training it to burn some of its fat stores.

Next, the body feels "sad" or deprived. Who wouldn't feel sad if you know you can't eat your favorite indulgences, even juts for a few hours and for your own good? Cravings are a way for the body to get that glucose hit. Studies found that certain types of sugars do trigger that area in the brain linked to addiction. Eating loads of sugar increases the level of certain happy hormones, making you feel good.

Cravings try to make you eat sugary foods to combat feelings of deprivation and sadness.

Not convinced?

Didn't you, at least once, ate an entire tub of ice cream or a big bag of chocolate chips or loads of chocolate éclairs when you felt sad?

Distract yourself when you feel cravings setting in. be busy. One great idea is to engage in exercise. You fight off cravings and reap the benefits of a good workout.

Do whatever you can to not think about food, and be sure to indulge a little during your feeding window so you have the chance to satisfy those cravings.

It's only temporary, as with most other side effects of the keto diet. Hang in there.

Irritability

Hangry is what this is. Feeling a little cranky is normal during the first few days. There's a lot going on in your body with all the fasting, glycogen depletion, dropping blood sugar levels, and fat burning going on.

To be less cranky, focus your energies into things that you enjoy. This way, you can also distract yourself from cravings.

Digestive issues

Heartburn, bloating, constipation, and diarrhea are part of the transition period of the digestive tract. Avoid this by drinking lots of water.

Heartburn comes from too much acid produced in the stomach. Since you won't be eating, this excess acid can produce heartburn. Over time, this will eventually go away. To keep heartburn from bothering you, drink lots of water. Sleep with your head propped. This will prevent the acid from flowing towards the esophagus. You can also help prevent severe heartburn by avoiding spicy and greasy foods during the eating window.

The most common cause of constipation is dehydration, although some people may experience this while adapting to fasting. Remember, you will be excreting lots fluids through the urine. One way to get through this is by adding more fiber into the diet. Eat more non-starchy vegetables. Add more salt for fluid balance. More importantly, stay hydrated. Drink lots of water. If these do not help relieve constipation, check your meals. Cut back on dairy and nuts. Taking 40 mg magnesium citrate may also help.

On the other hand, diarrhea may happen. This may happen during the first few days into the keto diet. This is, again, temporary. It's just part of the body's adjustment to the change in then macronutrient ratio of the meals. Some people think that diarrhea is a result of eating too much fats. This leads them to replace carbs with more proteins and reduce their fat intake. It's not the fats. It's just part of the transition period. To ease diarrhea, it would help to take psyllium husk powder, 1 teaspoon before meals. Taking sugar-free Metamucil can also help.

The digestive system will adjust to this change in diet.

Muscle Cramps

Some people may experience muscle cramps, especially in the legs. This is one of the side effects of losing fluids and minerals, especially potassium, during the initial phase.

To counter this, add more potassium-rich foods in meals. and adding more salt will help too. Drinking lots of water can also help to remove any lactic acid buildup that may be contributing to muscle cramps.

Supplements can also help. One recommended supplement is magnesium slow-release tablets. Take 3 tablets daily for 20 days. After that, reduce magnesium dose to once daily.

Sleep Disturbances

Sometimes, going to sleep may be a little more difficult during the initial stage of the Keto OMAD diet. This is due to lower levels of insulin occurring with lower levels of serotonin.

To help with this side effect, eat a small protein-rich snack before going to bed. The snack should also contain a small amount of carbohydrates as this will help raise insulin levels resulting in more tryptophan to the brain. Tryptophan is a precursor of serotonin which means that boosting tryptophan results in increased serotonin production.

Another potential reason for sleep troubles is eating foods rich in histamines. Some fat-rich, protein-rich foods are also high in histamines. These foods include bacon, eggs, avocados and cheeses.

If you have trouble sleeping, you may omit these foods from your diet at least temporarily. Replace these with added servings of vegetables.

Smelly Breath

Smelly breath is more appropriately called acetone breath, it is sometimes also referred to as "keto breath". This is caused by increased levels of ketones in the body. Ketones give off that fruity acetone smell similar to the smell of nail polish remover.

Having acetone breath is actually a good sign. It means that the body is converting more fats and producing adequate amounts of ketones. It means you really are ketogenic state.

This smell will eventually go away once the body has already adapted to ketosis. This will usually take about 1-2 weeks.

Smelly acetone breath is not serious. However, this can be a cause of concern as nobody wants to smell bad.

To improve the smell, try these tips:

- Maintain good oral hygiene. Brush the teeth at 2 times daily.

- Drink more water. Dry mouth worsens bad breath. On a low-carb diet, the body release water and can lead to less saliva, resulting in dry mouth.

- Breath fresheners. It may not totally mask the fruity acetone smell but it can help reduce that smell.

It may help to slightly increase the carb content of meals. However, defer this for a few more weeks. Allow the body time to adjust and the smell naturally goes away. Do not make adjustments to carb contents just to remove bad breath. If after a few weeks the smell does not go away, add more carbs 50 to 70 grams a day.

What about staying in ketosis?

The fasting window of OMAD should help keep you in ketosis even with the increased carb intake.

Palpitations

People who have normally lower blood pressures have greater chances of experiencing increased heart palpitations. This is more likely from loss of fluids and electrolytes.

Again, during the first few days of ketosis, fluids and electrolytes are removed from the body through increased urination. This results in lower circulating blood volume. In response, the heart tries to compensate by pumping harder, in an attempt to supply enough blood, oxygen and nutrients to the tissues.

Again, this is nothing to be worried about. Heart palpitations go away on its own as the body adjusts to ketosis. It should be gone by week 1 to week2 on the keto diet.

If heart palpitations persist, increasing carb intake can help. To keep the keto benefits, the OMAD diet with an 8-hour eating window (that includes increased carb intake) can help.

Taking supplements can also help such as high quality multivitamin supplements that contain selenium and zinc. Taking magnesium supplements also helps by replacing lost nutrients during the transition period.

However, people with cardiovascular problems will have to work with their doctors. Heart palpitations in these people are not to be taken lightly.

Flu Symptoms

When on the Keto OMAD diet, it is common to feel like you are coming down with the flu during the first week into the diet. Symptoms like lethargy, headaches, tiredness, and irritability are very common. Some people may even experience confusion or what they describe as a "brain fog".

This is normal. This phenomenon is called "Keto Flu" or "Induction Flu", which is your body's adaptation from burning sugars to burning fats for energy. Fasting may also trigger these symptoms as well as your body adapts from eating multiple meals a day to only eating one meal a day.

Whether your symptoms are brought about by the keto flu or adjustment from fasting, it is the result of lower insulin levels and dropping blood sugar levels. Obviously, eating carbs will make you feel better but that would break your fast, and kick you out of ketosis. So what can you do if you don't want to drop your diet?

The answer is simple: drink water and stay hydrated. Increasing your salt intake and getting enough fats can also help improve your condition dramatically. Make sure you get enough sleep, too. The body will have a lot of resting and recuperating to do at this time.

You might also want to try to schedule your days to be more relaxing. Fasts should be scheduled when you won't have to do too many things during the day.

CHAPTER 6

What and When to Eat on the Keto OMAD Diet

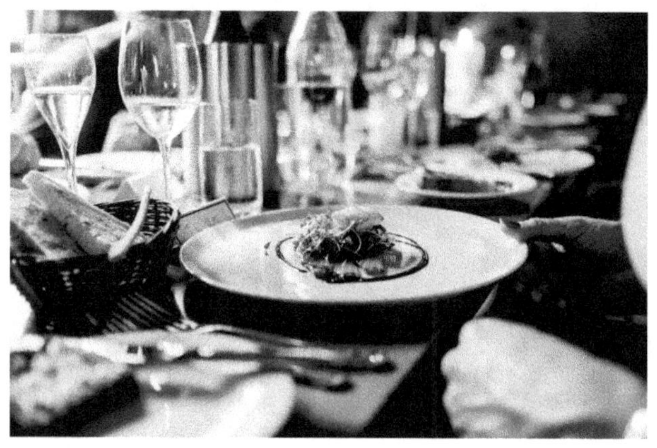

The key to the success of the Keto OMAD diet is eating small amounts of carbohydrates and high in fats and proteins. There are also few other guidelines to follow to handle the side effects, avoid mistakes and reap optimum benefits which have been covered in earlier chapters.

What to Eat on the Keto OMAD Diet

So what do you eat on the Keto OMAD diet?

Think of all carbohydrate-rich foods and say goodbye to them. That includes pasta and rice, plus bread and noodles. Starchy vegetables are out, too. That will essentially be removing most of what an average person eats every day. So what food is left?

If you're thinking you will be depriving yourself of all the good foods out there, think again. There are still tons of delicious, filling foods out there that conform to your new diet. In fact, you may find yourself enjoying the keto food list better than your previous unhealthy meals.

Foods to include would be:

Seafood

These are rich, delicious protein sources but low in carbs and high in healthy fats. Fish and seafood are also high in minerals like selenium, potassium and B vitamins. Most of these are also carb-free.

However, there are a few that may have higher carbohydrate contents. Take a look at these examples:

- Mussels: 7 grams carbs

- Clams: 5 grams

- Oysters: 4 grams

- Octopus: 4 grams

- Squid: 3 grams

Some of the top choices for fishes for keto meals are high in omega-3 fats. This includes salmon, mackerel and sardines. These help lower levels of insulin and improve insulin sensitivity, especially in overweight and obese people.

The recommendation is eating at least 2 fish servings per week.

Low carb veggies

Some veggies are high in carbs, which you should avoid to maintain ketosis. Aim to add more low carb veggies as these are rich in vitamins and minerals to help balance the body's many cellular processes. Also, add more veggies that are in fiber. This helps you feel full and improve the satiety of your meals. It also helps counteract constipation induced by eating lots of fats and proteins.

These non-starchy vegetables have low net carbs. That means the amount carbs that the body actually absorbs and turned into glucose. The calories may be high in these vegetables but if you subtract the fiber contents, the net carbs will mean you only get to absorb small amounts. Fiber is counted towards the carbohydrate count of food. However, it is not digested and absorbed. Hence, it can be removed from the total carb content.

One impact of eating these kinds of vegetables is that you do provide your body with enough calories but you only get to absorb a small amount of carbohydrates that get turned into glucose.

To make choosing much easier, most vegetables that grow above ground are low in carbs so add them in your meals. Examples are broccoli, cabbage, and leafy greens.

Those that grow underground are typically starchy ones so avoid these. Examples to avoid are potatoes and beets.

Cheese

Do not be afraid of eating cheese. It is high in fats and low in carbs. Plus, it is a good source of calcium.

Some are hesitant about eating cheese because of its high saturated fats content. The kind of saturated fats in cheeses do not contribute to higher risk for heart diseases. They may even help protect the cardiovascular system against diseases.

Avocados

It is high in fats that can help you feel full longer. It may be high in calories, at 9 grams for a 100-gram serving of avocado. However, 7 grams of these is fiber. Therefore, you may eat 9 grams carbohydrates but your body may inly absorb up to 2 grams.

Poultry, Meats

These are staples on the ketogenic diet. These are high in fats and proteins without any carbs. It also has B vitamins and minerals such as zinc, potassium and selenium.

Choose grass-fed meats and poultry as these have more omega-3 fats compared to commercially-raised animals.

Eggs

Eggs are high in fats with moderate amounts of proteins. These have many vitamins and minerals, with less than 1 gram of carbohydrates.

These are perfect for the keto lifestyle.

These are also very versatile and easy to cook. A large batch of scrambled eggs is easy to cook, even when you are rushing in the morning. They pack in a lots of fats that make you feel full until non or even later in the afternoon.

Coconut oil

It's a healthy kind of oil that contains MCTs (medium-chain triglycerides). If you're on a keto diet, MCTs are very helpful. They speed up the time it takes for the body to reach ketosis.

Olive oil

Like coconut oil, olive oil is also beneficial for the heart. It has monounsaturated fats that reduce the risk for developing cardiovascular problems such as heart attacks and stroke.

Olive oil is also rich in phenols. These are compounds that reduce inflammation, thereby reducing risk for heart problems.

Seeds, Nuts

These are low in carbs and high in fats. Plus, they add some nice texture to foods.

Nuts and seeds also pack in lots of fiber. These can help improve heart health, keep you full and reduce risk for chronic diseases.

Some of the good nuts and seeds for keto meals include:

- Brazil nuts: 3 grams total carbs (1 gram net carbs)
- Pecans: 4 grams total carbs (1 gram net carbs)
- Macadamia nuts: 4 grams total carbs (2 grams net carbs)
- Walnuts: 4 grams total carbs (2 grams net carbs)
- Almonds: 6 grams total carbs (3 grams net carbs)
- Flaxseeds: 8 grams total carbs (0 grams net carbs)
- Chia seeds: 12 grams total carbs (1 gram net carbs)

Berries

Tart berries have lower sugar content and high antioxidant content. Examples of these berries include blueberries and blackberries. The antioxidants help protect the body from free radical damage and reduce inflammation.

Some berries may be high in calories but are high in fiber.

Cream, Butter

These are easy ingredients that can add more fats into your meals to maintain ketosis. These have been considered by many in the past years to be bad food because of high saturated fat contents. The saturated fats in these foods are not liked to increased risk for heart diseases.

Others

Other keto-friendly foods include:

- Olives
- Unsweetened Coffee and Tea
- Bone broth
- Dark Chocolate and Cocoa Powder
- Natural fat, high-fat sauces

<u>*What foods to avoid*</u>

The list of foods to avoid on ketogenic diet is much shorter. Just remove anything high in carbs and you're good. You will have to avoid:

- Whole grains
- Milk
- Chicken nuggets
- Cold cuts
- Dried fruits
- Ice cream
- Desserts
- Alcohol

When to Eat on the Keto OMAD Diet

The OMAD portion of the Keto OMAD requires that you have a four hour window to eat one meal a day as part of the 4 "Ones" so when is the best time for you to have your meal?

The simple answer is "whenever it is most convenient for you".

Some people choose to skip two meals and only eat either breakfast or dinner. Others just grab their meal whenever they have an opening in their schedule. There are also people who practice fasting by listening to their body, skipping meals if they don't feel hungry. This works only if your body has already been conditioned to live on irregular food schedules.

The only time where there is a consideration to be made is when exercise is involved.

When you exercise on any form of fasting diet, you should consume something half an hour after your workout session. Remember that you don't have to strictly stay on OMAD if it makes sense for you not to fast for the day.

There are also people who only fast on alternate days, or on weekends. The crucial thing is that you have make your diet fit your lifestyle and be consistent with it in order for OMAD to work.

The Secret to Making the Keto OMAD Diet Work

Diets usually focus on the foods that you can or cannot eat in order to maintain a calorie deficit. The idea is that if your body burns more energy than it takes in, you will lose weight. However, this works against your body as it leads you to take food that is low in nutritional value. If you are not satisfied with your meal, it leaves you hungry.

Research has also found that reducing food intake can increase your risk of binge eating as it prompts your brain to develop cravings. The more you deny yourself food, the more you are likely to end up wanting to eat. Therefore, planning your meals is important. Having evenly spaced meals at regular intervals allows your stomach to produce ghrelin at the appropriate times to adjust to your meal patterns.

When you are used to eating every few hours or so, your stomach is trained to send hunger signals at regular intervals. This is why you should figure out a schedule that works best for you and try to stick with it as much as possible, factoring in adjustments to your schedule.

A waiting period between meals is also necessary to give time for your previous meal to move to the small intestine. This helps to ensure that your appetite is "real" and you are not eating out of habit or eating as an emotional response. This may also result in problems for your blood sugar as the glucose from your second meal spikes while the glucose from your first meal is still in your bloodstream.

CHAPTER 7

Whole Foods vs. Processed Foods

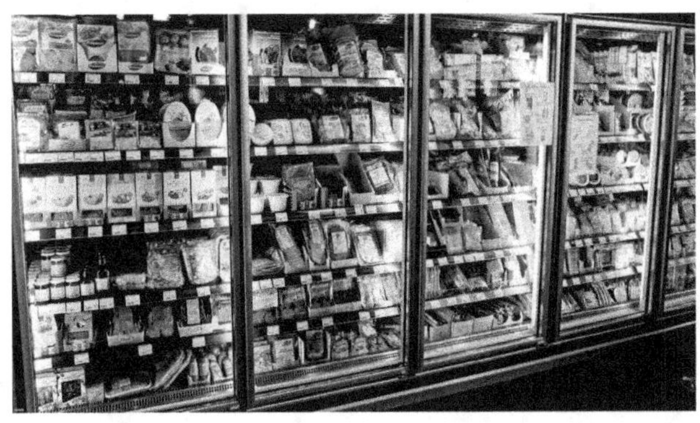

Before we get into planning your diet and lifestyle, I would like to take a chapter to discuss th spectrum of food. At one end are the healthiest options, these are whole foods. At the other end are highly processed foods which are unhealthy.

Let us look into the type of foods available in the market and how they make a difference to your diet and your nutrition.

Unprocessed Foods

Processed foods are foods that have been frozen, canned, dried, or otherwise preserved after cooking. They have their natural composition altered in some way.

These are not limited to just microwaveable frozen meals or canned meals and can include items such as:

- Canned fruit and vegetables
- Cookies
- Chips and crackers
- Cheese
- Bacon, ham, sausages, and other deli meats
- Bottled or packet sauces
- Instant ramen
- Dried fruit and fruit snacks

When food is pre-packaged or processed are produced, the goal is to have the best possible shelf life and yet maintain its taste and flavor. To do this, the preserving process involves the use of preservatives to extend the shelf life, sugars and salt is used to enhance the taste, and food coloring is used to make it look tasty despite being kept for long periods.

Even sliced fruits and vegetables that are processed are not healthy options. Fresh fruit and vegetables oxidize in minutes. Leave a slice of apple out in the open and you will see it start to turn brown but soak it in salt water and it stays looking fresh for a longer period. Imagine how much salt or sugar you would need to keep it looking fresh for hours, days, or even months. Chemicals such as copper sulfate, rhodamine oxide, malachite green and carbide, which can be deadly, are often added to accentuate the color and freshness of these processed fruits. Some of these chemicals are derived from oils, and others may penetrate deep inside the food. When that happens it is not easily washed away and we unknowingly consume them.

In short, the issue with processed foods is that we have no control over the amount of salt, sugar, fats, and chemicals that goes into our diet when we eat them. These heavily processed foods and drinks promote weight gain and obesity and increases our risk for diabetes, cardiovascular disease, as well as cancer.

Whole Foods

Aside from avoiding or reducing your intake of processed foods, a healthier choice to make would be replace the processed foods with whole foods. These are foods that are close to their natural state. These would usually be located at the fresh section of your grocery store or supermarket.

You should choose fresh fruit, vegetables, and meat instead of frozen, canned, or dried options where possible. If it comes in a foil bag, a cardboard box, a plastic tray, or a can it is usually not as nutritious as the "loose" pieces of fruit, vegetables, or meat.

While high sugar and high salt foods that are processed can be filling, it does have an effect on your blood sugar, your blood pressure, your cholesterol, and your insulin levels. Whole foods, however, retain their fiber as well as their nutrients especially phytochemicals.

Phytochemicals are bioactive nonnutrient plant compounds that are found in fruit, grain, and vegetables. These have been found to reduce the risk of chronic diseases and may even prevent heart disease and cancer. There are studies dating as far back as 2003 have shown that they provide massive health benefits as well.

Whole foods are also rich in vitamins, fiber, and potassium as well as healthy fats that benefit your HDL cholesterol levels. So aside from avoiding high amounts of salt, sugar and chemicals in processed foods, replacing them with whole foods provides more benefits to your overall health and wellbeing. Additionally, whole foods help you with weight loss as they provide satiety and make you feel full with less calories.

Whole foods help you with weight loss because they usually contain less calories per gram than processed foods. This is because they have more water and a high fiber content. This difference means that you decrease the amount of calories you absorb per serving of whole food as compared to processed foods since your body has to work harder to digest and assimilate the nutrients.

The 3 main ingredients added to processed foods, namely fat, sugar, and salt, have been found to stimulate our taste buds and leave us craving for more. A study published in PLOS One in 2013 has linked overeating to the high amounts of refined sugar and fat in diets. By switching to whole foods we reduce the fat, sugar, and salt that we consume which helps us to prevent overeating as well.

CHAPTER 8

Planning Your Diet

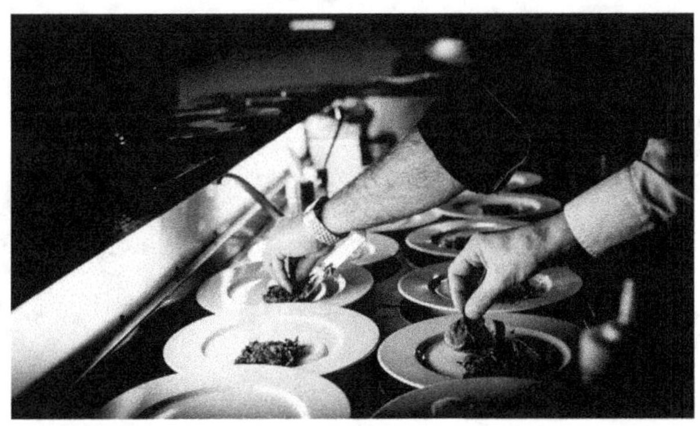

Both diets come with discomfort as these promote a drastic change in the body. Fasting places the body in a state that uses glycogen and fat stores by not eating for extended periods. Keto diet drastically reduces carbohydrate intake and replacing most of the day's calorie sources to fats.

To ease the discomforts and hurdle through the challenges of both diets, _start with keto diet first_.

When your body is used to having carbohydrates as an energy source you very likely will be used to eating a lot and frequently throughout the day. This will mean that you will get hungry faster than when you are keto adapted.

When you are in ketosis and using ketones for energy, it will be easier to stick to your fasting schedule. This can be a more comfortable transition than racing headlong into fasting. Fasting immediately without proper preparation can make it harder to stick to the diet.

By starting with keto, the body is slowly conditioned to look for other energy sources other than carbs. This way, once you go introduce fasting into your lifestyle, the body is no longer too dependent on glucose. By this time, it will be used to using fats/ketones.

To start the keto diet:

- Remove all carbohydrate-rich foods in the pantry. Remove all processed foods and junk foods as well.

- List down the fat-rich foods included in the keto diet.

- Shop for good fats such as olive oil, sesame oil and butter.

- Replace meals with keto meals. This can be as simple as removing pasta and eating steak with marinara sauce, eat burgers without the buns or removing toast and eat more eggs instead for breakfast.

Follow the keto diet for about 3 days or so, to get things going. It does take that long to put the body into true ketosis.

Ease into fasting and eventually OMAD. It is suggested that before you cut to one meal a day it is advisable to practice a less demanding fasting routine first.

At this stage, you should start cutting your meals and make it a point that you should end the eating window with a keto meal. Your last meal before you start the fast is just as important as the fast itself. This will feed the body and prepare it for the changes that will happen.

Eat a keto meal. If you are starting the fast before bedtime, eat a keto-rich meal such as a good juicy steak with butter and a good helping of fiber-rich, low-carbohydrate salad such as asparagus sautéed in butter or roasted with olive oil.

If you are fasting during the daytime, aim for a keto breakfast. Try almond flour muffins with butter, bacon and scrambled eggs. Skip lunch and dinner. This schedule is good for those who want to go on a 24-hour fast. A small serving of bone broth before bedtime can help ease hunger and promote better sleep. It is difficult to sleep on an empty stomach.

These recommendations are helpful in getting results fast. Keto diet will start putting the body into ketosis. Once fasting starts, this effect will be complemented by autophagy.

Together, these two processes will bring the desired benefits in no time. Spend 3 days on keto diet before starting to fast. This not only helps prepare your body better for the rigors of fasting, it will also help reduce keto flu.

Things to Keep in Mind on Keto OMAD

The start of a new diet is usually the hardest part. Here are some quick tips to make your diet easier.

Take MCT Oil Before Your Fast

MCT or medium-chain triglycerides oil promotes the release of peptide YY and leptin; these two hormones help with satiety. Meaning you feel full for longer. These oils are also easily broken down in the body making them easily absorbed in your digestive system.

There are some studies that shown that MCT oils prevent obesity and reduce weight, but there are also reports otherwise. The Journal of Nutrition published a paper in 2002 that showed MCT oil raised the metabolic rate of the participants of the study. However the effect was really small. 5 grams of MCT oil was found to burn an extra 11 calories a day.

MCT oil can be can be found in coconut oil, butter, milk, yogurt, and cheese.

It is frequently added into keto meals to speed up ketone production. People who fast take it before a fast helps to reach a state of ketosis faster, and if you're already in ketosis it helps you to stay in ketosis. This helps to get optimum benefits from the fast within a shorter period.

MCT oil will break your fast, so the best time to take it is right before you start the fast. On a Keto OMAD diet, that usually means that you should consume MCT oil during your meal if possible.

Take Lots of Electrolytes

The keto diet is diuretic, meaning that it causes you to pass a lot of urine. This can be a problem because it could cause you to lose electrolytes. These are minerals in your body that contain an electric charge and they help to balance the water in your body and move nutrients and wastes around to the appropriate place.

When you are low on electrolytes, it will cause symptoms such as irregular heartbeat, fatigue, lethargy, nausea, and vomiting among others. These are typically known as the "keto flu". Taking an electrolyte drink, or sports drink, can replace these electrolytes. Just remember to choose one that does not have sugar.

Stay Hydrated

Drink lots of water on Keto OMAD. "Keto breath" from acetones is a common side effect of the keto diet and water helps to treat that.

Drinking lots of water also helps with hunger pangs that commonly occurs when fasting, especially longer fasts like OMAD. Very often, when we feel hungry it might be thirst instead.

Common symptoms of keto and OMAD such as fatigue, headaches, and nausea can also be caused by dehydration.

Plan Ahead

When starting out on Keto, it helps to be prepared. Stock up your pantry and fridge with staples that you need. These are foods like your meat, eggs, cheese, butter, avocados, spinach, and nuts. You would also want to consume or dispose of your non keto food beforehand so you don't risk eating something that breaks you out of ketosis.

On the topic of planning ahead, you may also want to consider prepping your meals. Thinking about what dishes to cook and what meats, veggies, and other foods you need will help you to meet your daily nutrient goals.

Since the fasting window on OMAD is pretty long, having prepped meals helps to shorten your cooking times. Trust me, you will be hungry and might be tempted to cut corners when mealtime comes around. Planning ahead helps you ensure your meals are tasty, nutritious, and best of all, easily accessible when you need them.

Start Slow

Once your body adapts to burning fat, you will naturally feel hungry less often. As a result you will find that you can easily skip meals and cut your carb intake. It is recommended that you start with the keto diet simply because it is the easier adjustment of the two diets.

Once you have successfully transitioned to a keto diet, then you can take the next step by cutting out snacks. By passing on snacks that could easily be an extra 1000 calories a day that we're avoiding. The final step is to start fasting by skipping one meal a day, or restricting your eating window. From there you can more easily adjust from two meals to one meal a day.

As with any diet, remember that this is a marathon and not a sprint. There is little point in starving yourself for a week or even a month. The idea is to comfortably have a schedule that you can manage. What that is may look different for all of us.

CHAPTER 9

Working Out on Keto OMAD

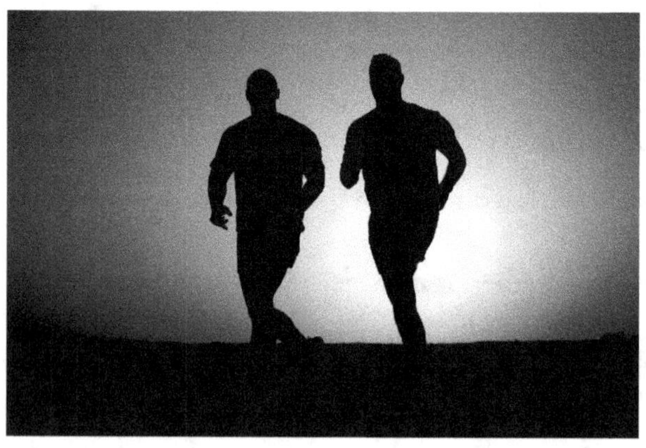

Gaining muscle mass is not impossible, but much harder with a ketogenic diet. Fasting solves this by improving the body's insulin sensitivity, blood glucose regulation, and human growth hormone (HGH) production with helps to boost muscle growth.

The HGH is also known as the "exercise hormone" as well as the "fitness hormone". It increases our muscle growth and improves our performance when working out. By burning body fat, HGH production is increased.

Fasting for 24 hours reduces your insulin levels. Insulin levels has been shown from research to disrupt HGH production. After fasting for three days HGH levels can increase by up to 300%, and after a week it can increase by up to 1,250%.

When working out, your adrenaline levels rise. Together with the production of HGH and lowering of insulin resistance, this combination starts fat breakdown (adipose tissue lipolysis) and fat burning for energy (peripheral fat oxidation).

There are many studies that have shown that exercising in a fasted state helps to body to adapt to glycogen depletion which increases fat loss by up to 20 percent. This is because when we are not fasted, insulin is increased in our body, and higher insulin levels are linked with a slow-down of fat burning metabolism by the same amount of approximately 20 percent.

This basically means that exercising on an empty stomach makes our bodies more efficient at using fat rather than sugar as fuel giving us a better result for our effort.

If you add ketosis, you can increase the benefits you get from exercise. Ketosis further supports fat burning. It also helps improve insulin function.

What Happens When You Fast and Exercise?

The Standford University School of Medicine has shown that diet and exercise have a synergistic relationship; they both help your weight loss. Diet restricts your caloric intake and increases your intake of valuable nutrients, and exercise helps to burn calories as well as build lean muscle mass. Building muscle will help to burn more calories while at rest.

On the OMAD diet, when we are in a fasted state our bodies start to use our stored fat and glycogen reserves as its main energy source to provide energy for our daily activities.

But what about when you exercise while you are in a fasted state?

A 2009 study showed that carbohydrate restriction through intermittent fasting, when coupled with exercise, can increase the endurance among trained athletes.

Exercising with low glycogen in our bodies also increases the mitochondrial biogenesis, which is the process wherein new mitochondria are formed within the cells. Mitochondria provide more energy to sustain individual cells during the workout and are known as the powerhouse of the cell.

Lastly, when working in a fasted state, the preservation mechanism of the body that protects active muscles are activated. This prevents active muscles from wasting away, which is known as muscle atrophy. Therefore, we are effectively burning our fat and glycogen stores instead of muscles contrary to popular belief.

Remember those exercise routines burn energy that supports weight loss and training under a fasted state provides some unique benefits in terms of fat loss.

How Ketosis Impacts Exercise Performance

When our bodies don't have access to glycogen it loses some of its ability to function under maximum effort. Fat and ketones does not replace glucose in the glycolytic pathway. This means that when you go all out for more than 10 seconds, and less than 120 seconds it must be fueled by glucose. After 120 seconds, your body starts to shift to a metabolic pathway that burns ketones and fats.

In simple terms, this means that when our bodies are in ketosis our performance is limited for high intensity exercises such as lifting heavy weights or when doing circuit training. In fact, when on the Keto OMAD diet it is not recommended that you do any vigorous exercise. It does not, however, affect your performance on endurance activities such as cycling or jogging.

On the positive side however, ketosis can help to burn more fat. A study on ultra-endurance runners published in 2016 found that those on a low carb diet burned up to three times as much fat during a three hour run as compared to those on a high carb diet. There was also no difference in the amount of muscle glycogen used between both groups, meaning that there was no loss of muscle.

A study published in 2009 has shown that eating a low carb high fat diet does not have an effect on your exercise performance. This process is called keto-adaptation.

Keto-adaptation means that your body gets more efficient at using ketones as fuel, and usually takes place after a few weeks on a ketogenic diet. This is when your body makes gradual changes such as conserving protein, and reducing the lactic acid buildup after working out. This means you feel less fatigued and sore from exercise.

Macros for Your Keto OMAD Workouts

On any ketogenic diet, your macros are very important. Keeping the right balance of *fats*, *proteins*, and *carbs* helps your body function optimally. When you add a work out to the equation, managing your macros becomes even more important.

The Keto OMAD diet cuts calories by restricting carbs. It is the lack of carbs that puts you into ketosis after all. Add to that the appetite suppressing effect of high protein and high fat in your diet, and you could be under eating especially if you take into account the additional demands that working out places on your body.

Since carbs help to preserve muscle stimulus, when it is absent or lacking in our diet (because of keto), we need to use fat and protein to maintain performance and gain muscle mass. Therefore, having the right amount of fat and protein is more important when exercising in a state of ketosis.

Protein is vitally important when working out on the Keto OMAD diet. Protein improves your satiation. But more importantly, protein helps to build muscle, prevents muscle loss, and burns more calories than fats and carbs.

Fats are just as important on the keto diet. There is a common misconception that keto is about eating meat. Having a high protein, low carb, and low fat diet can actually lower your muscle mass because you don't have enough fat to compensate for the carbs that you have cut. As a result, you may not actually be in ketosis.

Lastly, the quality of your food is just as important as the quantity. Eating fresh, whole foods would provide more nutrients than canned or processed foods even if the protein and fat is the same. This is because the canning process and preservatives added are used to keep the food looking fresh. Frozen dinners are convenient and tasty, but are lacking in nutrients and vitamins.

Protein when Working Out on Keto OMAD

Protein is what is known as a "macronutrient" or a "macro" for short. Unlike vitamins and minerals, we need a comparatively larger amount of it.

Research has shown that meals that are higher in protein improve satiety and make you feel fuller. This is attributed to protein triggering a release of certain gut hormones that are responsible for making you feel full by sending signals to your brain. Comparatively, these hormones are not released in such high quantities when you consume fat or carbohydrates.

This appetite suppressing function of protein is also directly proportional to the amount of protein consumed. Meaning that people who consume more protein as a percentage of their diet tend to feel full faster. As a result they have lower amounts of abdominal fat as they feel full eating less calories.

In a study by the International Society of Sports Nutrition, researchers found that a protein intake of 0.6 grams to 0.9 grams per pound (1.4 grams to 2 grams per kilogram) of lean body mass is ideal amount for people who exercise regularly.

Bodybuilders have a rule of thumb where they take 1 gram of protein per pound of their body weight. When trying to lose fat, some bodybuilders can increase that ratio to 1.5 grams per pound. This is also recommended on the Keto OMAD diet as it will help preserve muscle mass; just be sure to increase your fat intake in your diet accordingly.

There is also another benefit from the increased protein because your body will use it for gluconeogenesis. This is when your muscles use the non carbohdrate nutrients to maintain your blood glucose levels.

CONCLUSION

Thank you for taking the time to read this book!

The OMAD diet and ketogenic diet is a powerful combination when put together. Each complements the benefits of the other while helping to address the side effects and risks.

There are many who have gone through this program and gained many benefits, including a more sustainable and easier to maintain weight loss.

However, this is not a one-size-fits-all kind of weight loss program. People with serious health conditions or existing high risk for chronic diseases are highly advised to work closely with their doctors to go on OMAD and ketogenic diet.

The next step here is to consult with your doctor and a fitness instructor, begin planning your meals and workouts, and starting on your journey. If you can, take action today; the longer you put things off the more likely you are to continue procrastinating.

With that said, I hope you learned a lot from this book. Apply the concepts discussed here and see for yourself how much OMAD and keto diet can do for you.

Train safe, eat healthy, and and best wishes for you fitness and weight loss journey!